The Alzheimer's and Vascular Dementia Disease Diet

By
Lynne D M Noble

Copyright 2019 Lynne D M Noble

Independently published

Dedication

To Vera Xx

About the Author

Lynne Noble was born in 1953 in Huddersfield, West Yorkshire. From a very early age, Lynne showed an interest in nutrition and genetics avidly reading any books that she could get her hands on at the time.

Initially, Lynne studied orthopaedics but events led her to work with the elderly mentally infirm. Here, her interest in neurodegenerative disorders and pain syndromes developed.

Lynne undertook rigorous programmes of study, completing her Cert Ed., (FE) BSc (Hons) and Adv. Dip Education simultaneously before moving onto her M.Ed.

From there she took further demanding programmes in Human Nutrition, Pharmacology, Neuroscience, Genetics and Immunology. During this time, she was given many prestigious awards for her academic work. It was noted then that Lynne was not afraid of tackling difficult subjects.

She began her law degree but ill health prevented her from pursuing this. However, in this time, she moved from being a foster parent to adoptive parent.

She has been instrumental in setting up projects in the community for disadvantaged groups.

She is a member of the Guild of Health Writers.

Now retired, she lives in a picturesque village in West Yorkshire with her husband. She enjoys gardening, watching her husband bowling and researching.

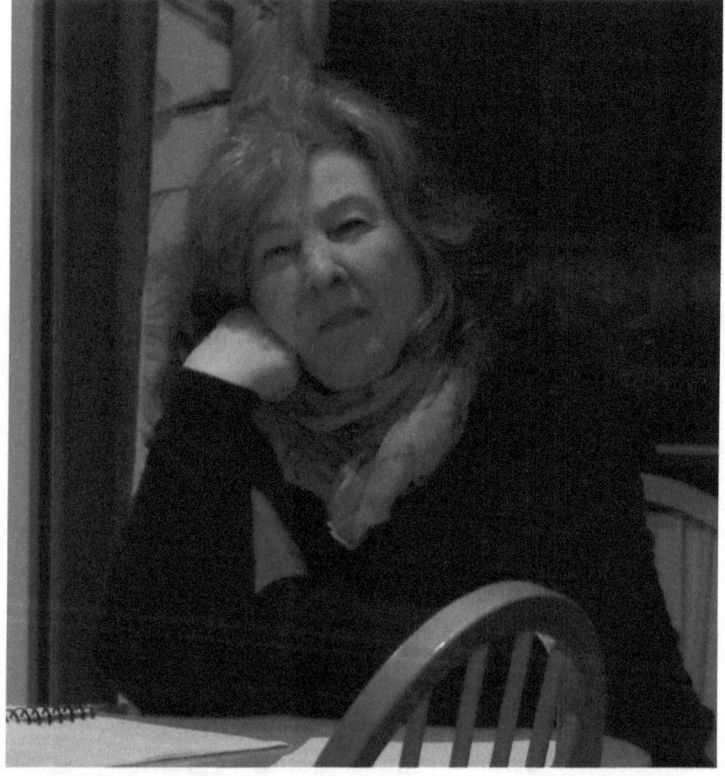

Author Lynne Noble at home

https://quintessentiallylynne.weebly.com/nutritional-medicine.html

Fragility wraps itself around her

Like a dying breath composed of pale hues

And longing that the time of departure

Will be stayed, yet knowing it will not.

For life is ever short,

Yet the pain of life much longer

But still, tis sweet

This life, made sweeter by its brevity.

Lynne D M Noble 2018

Dedication

To Vera – I wish I could have helped you more but what I have learned from the short time that I had with you, I will put to good use. Xx

Acknowledgement

There are probably far too many people who need acknowledging for inspiring me to write this book. I first had the idea to write this book when I had come across one too many people who had one of the dementias. Many were friends. I worked with people who had dementia. I observed, I researched and then I observed some more.

I was too young then to take what I had seen much further. There are rules you see. Rules that prevent us from asking questions when we are not wholly qualified to do so. Now that I am my questions or my observations or conclusions are not any different but now I am allowed to voice them.

When I look back it is Vera who sparked off my interest in looking further into the causes – and treatment - of Alzheimer's disease.   She will never know this because she was in the final stages of dementia when I came to know her but we 'met' briefly during the time that she lived in the residential home where I worked.

I wish that I had known then what I know now – Alzheimer's has not been around forever - it is a new disease that has been carved by our own unique set of environmental factors that impinge on genetic propensity.   Change or remove some of the offending environmental factors and the course of a disease can be changed.

Vera inadvertently taught me that.

Table of Contents

Preface

One of the greatest privileges I have had - once I moved from working in orthopaedics – was working in residential homes for the elderly. It did not take long before I came across residents with various forms of neurodegenerative disorder including Alzheimer's disease and the vascular dementias.

I was fortunate in that these conditions have not manifested themselves in either side of the family. We are a family blessed with longevity and you would think that the grasping fingers of dementia would touch a little part of some of us in some way in older age; more so as I know that the APOE E4 allele is found in both sides of the family.

The APOE E4 allele is a risk factor for Alzheimer's disease. However, I should hasten to add that a risk factor is not causation. It merely points to the fact, for whatever reason, that there appears to be a greater risk of being diagnosed with Alzheimer's disease if someone has one or both alleles. but it does not predict if and when this may occur. If a genetic predisposition is likely to unfold when you are 108 years old and you only live to 98 years of age, all is well and good in this matter.

Sometimes, a confused mind appears during times of infectious illness. A friend's husband became befuddled when he had a urine infection; my grandmother temporarily became confused when she had a respiratory infection. Both returned to full cognitive functioning once they had been treated with antibiotics. Why did this occur when it rarely happens in much younger people?

I know of people with marked neurofibrillary tangles and plaques who still play a full role in society and others with barely any tangles and plaques who are severely cognitively compromised. Why is this?

During my time at one residential home, I met 'Vera' who had had Alzheimer's for over five years. The staff could not cope with her for she did not have speech anymore and she could be quite violent and aggressive. I was quite intrigued by Vera as I am towards many whose behaviour will isolate them from others.

I made a point of sitting with her for half an hour over morning coffee and afternoon tea and just talking to her about everyday things. We sat away from the others where it was quiet. I did not get a response from her nor did I expect to. Nobody had ever heard Vera speak although her aggressive screaming was very much a part of what she had become. Still, when I spoke in our little enclave under the stairs, she became silent, sipping her coffee and nibbling on a biscuit. She only returned to marching up and down the corridors in a frenzied rage when our time together ended.

One afternoon when our afternoon tea date had finished, my shift happened to coincide with it.

'Well, Vera,' I said, 'my shift has ended and I am going home to my family now.'

Vera leaned over and placed a gnarled hand around my arm. 'Don't go.' She pleaded. 'Please don't go.'

Vera would not be consoled in spite of my promises that I would be back the following day. She followed me to the cloakroom and thereafter to the exit, not willing to let me go and it was only after some repeated promises that I would return, that eventually consoled her. If ever there was a lesson, that was it. A genetic condition may be present but by far the greatest factors in whether its potential is realised are the environmental ones. They are the greatest influence on any disease progression. Environmental factors include nutrition and social support but are not limited to these.

Good social support helps reduce the deterioration in communication and language skills that are symptomatic of the dementias. Loneliness is a terrible scourge on society and deterioration of cognitive functioning occurs rapidly in environments like this.

Nutrition is our biggest ally in the dementias. Good nutrition can change the course of a disease. It can slow its progression or stop it altogether. Sometimes it can reverse any damage that has been caused during the times when the disease process had been silently beginning to manifest itself in the body.

The fact that Alzheimer's disease and vascular dementia are generally a disease of older age gives us many clues as to the underlying processes that give rise to the symptoms. When those with diagnosed dementia are made temporarily worsened by a seemingly unrelated infection that gives us yet another clue as to the potential cause and remedy.

Diet does change the course of many diseases but there are never a one size fits all diet. A diet for iron deficiency anaemia is different from the diet to ameliorate the symptoms of diabetes type 2. Alzheimer's disease and vascular dementia are no different. They need bespoke diets to address the underlying pathological processes that are causing the symptoms.

This book is intended to do just that. It will show you which nutrients are vital for brain health and how they begin to address the underlying processes causing the conditions in the first place. It will show you which nutrients can help calm an overactive brain, reducing aggression and aiding sleep and which will help cognitive processing. There are even nutrients that have been shown to dissolve the amyloid beta plaques and remove them from brain to the blood. There are also nutrients that slow this process down and therefore contribute to the progression of dementia. It is not difficult to incorporate these nutrients into meals and requires only a few swaps of some foods, in other cases to provide brain friendly nutrients.

Although vascular dementia and Alzheimer's disease have some differences in aetiology there are also overlapping causative factors. Often individuals present with mixed dementia. This book is intended to not only address Alzheimer's and vascular dementia through diet but also has value for other neurodegenerative disorders.

As you read, you will begin to understand that our progressive healthy diets are not so healthy after all. In fact, the introduction of a few new healthy foods also coincided with the rise in Alzheimer's disease.

Supplementation of some vitamins and minerals is encouraged since it becomes harder to absorb nutrients as you get older and appetite is also much reduced making it harder to obtain the nutrients that you need for good brain health. A good multivitamin tablet would not go amiss although, even then, they generally do not contain 100% of the vitamins and mineral that particularly impact on brain health. However, they will go some way towards helping.

However, a word of caution here. Some trace metals, like copper, need to be bound to a protein. Without being bound, copper is toxic. The copper found in nutritional supplements, is unbound and has the potential to damage delicate brain tissue. It is better to avoid supplements that contain copper and obtain it from food where it will be bound to a protein source.

Dementia – some facts

Currently, 40.8 million people are living with dementia world-wide and this figure is expected to double approximately every twenty years so that in 2050 there are expected to be 115.4 million people worldwide suffering from some form of dementia.

Of these figures 17% of the above will be in the form of vascular dementia and another 10% will of mixed dementia that includes a combination of the underlying processes found in Alzheimer's disease and vascular dementia.

Vascular dementia

Vascular dementia occurs as a result of impaired blood flow. In many cases, a stroke may block an artery impeding the supply of nutrients and oxygen that the brain needs to function. However, other risk factors for vascular dementia include:

- High blood pressure
- Diabetes type II
- Smoking
- High cholesterol levels
- Atherosclerosis

We shall look at these in more detail later.

Unlike Alzheimer's disease which appears to have a pattern of steady decline, vascular dementia appears to have seven well documented stages of deterioration. Nevertheless, the symptoms include:

- Confusion
- Loss of attention and concentration
- A decline in ability to analyse situations effectively and to be able to communicate this effectively to others.
- Indecisiveness
- Inability to organise thoughts
- Difficulties with remembering
- Agitation
- Depression or apathy
- Incontinence
- Unsteady gait

Alzheimer's disease

Alzheimer's disease was first coined in 1906 by Alois Alzheimer who noted unusual behaviour in a mentally unstable lady. On her death, examination found amyloid plaques and tangled bundles of fibres known as neurofibrillary or tau tangles.

Tau proteins help stabilise microtubules that are abundant in the central nervous system. In Alzheimer's disease certain enzymes called tau kinases act on the tau protein. As a result, it becomes misfolded and clumps together. It has now become a neurofibrillary tangle. These tangles affect learning and memory.

Amyloid plaques are protein fragments. They are sticky plaques of beta amyloid. There is often a build-up of beta amyloid in those with Alzheimer's disease.

Plaques and tangles are considered to be the main features of Alzheimer's disease although that cannot be the whole story since many patients with marked tau tangles and plaques do not show symptoms of the disease. Others with relatively few changes can be grossly symptomatic of the disease. Nevertheless, those individuals with Down's Syndrome have a greatly increased risk for Alzheimer's disease. This is thought to be because they have an extra chromosome 21 and it is this chromosome that generates amyloid protein.

Ten years before symptoms show, there is believed to be a pre-clinical stage for Alzheimer's disease. This is characterised by the abnormal protein deposits found in amyloid plaques as well neurofibrillary tangles. Even at this stage healthy neurons stop functioning and begin to lose their connections. This initially occurs in the hippocampus and entorhinal cortex. These are parts of the brain that form memories. Eventually the disease process spreads out and the brain tissue begins to shrink.

Diagram showing hippocampus and entorhinal cortex

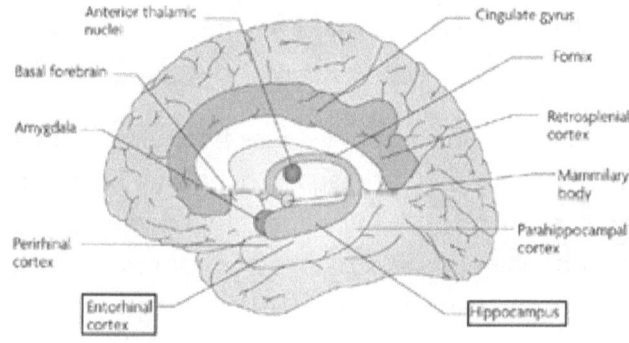

1

Potential Causes of Dementia

Low grade inflammation Is responsible for many of the chronic diseases that are now rife in society. When we think of chronic diseases and the vascular damage that they can do, then inflammation, caused by free radical damage production, springs to mind easily.

Inflammation, free radicals and antioxidants

Free radicals are everywhere; we can't avoid them. They are generated from the metabolism of food that we eat and they are generated from:

- Cigarette smoke
- Cosmetics
- Air pollution
- Pesticides
- Radiation

Indeed, anything that involves chemicals including household cleaners and perfumes.

Free radicals are unpaired electrons. Electrons are stable when paired up but if they are unpaired or odd they form free radicals. They are formed when oxygen interacts with certain molecules. Like an out of control pinball free radicals dash around damaging anything that they come into contact with. When they crash into important cellular components such as cell membranes or DNA then serious damage or cell death can occur.

Free radical damage can be risk factors for:

- Arthritis
- Cataracts
- The acceleration of the ageing process
- Some cancers
- Neurodegenerative disorders such as motor neuron disease, Parkinson's disease, vascular dementia and Alzheimer's disease

Antidotes to free radicals are antioxidants. Antioxidants are found in food but not the overcooked processed food that is often served up nowadays. When food is cooked most of the antioxidants are reduced or destroyed altogether. This does not mean that processed food does not have some benefit. It can still provide fibre, carbohydrates, fats, protein and some minerals. However, for the purposes of neutralising free radicals they do not offer much benefit for any neurodegenerative disease.

Antioxidants have to been taken in larger quantities than free radicals are being generated if we are to avoid the preclinical stages of dementia or slow down the progression of a degenerative disorder. This sounds difficult. We can make a guess that if the amount of processed food that we eat outweighs the non-processed food that we are not achieving our objective. However, we also have to take into consideration the external sources of free radicals such as household cleaners. We can now see that there is not much room for including processed food into the diet if we are trying to avoid damage to the cells and organs of our body.

Genetic propensity will play a role in which part of the body is most likely to be affected by free radicals.

There are a number of antioxidants that appear to have superior properties. These antioxidants are either minerals or vitamins.

Vitamins can be subdivided into fat soluble vitamins and water soluble and it is useful to understand their different properties before we embark further towards a bespoke diet for dementia.

The water soluble vitamins

The water soluble vitamins are the B and C vitamins. Vitamin C is probably one of the most well-known of the vitamins and most people know that it can be found in fresh fruit and vegetables. It is easily destroyed by heat whether this is by sunlight or cooking. As it is water soluble it easily leaches into the water that it is being cooked in. Any vitamin C that survives in the water is normally thrown away.

Vitamin C is a water soluble antioxidant and helps protect against cardiovascular disease and plaque formation. As such it has benefit for the dementias that are the subject matter of this book. We will look further at its properties when we discuss vitamin E which is a fat soluble vitamin.

Vitamin B forms part of a complex. There is vitamin B1, B2, B3, B5, B6, B9 and B12. They each have their own individual names such as riboflavin and thiamine. As water soluble vitamins they also leach into water and are easily destroyed.

An adequate supply of these vitamins needs to be ingested daily since any vitamin that is not required for immediate use is passed out of the body in urine.

Vitamin B12 is unusual in that it requires an acidic environment in order for it to be separated from its food source. The stomach acid of elderly people tends to be reduced and further, many elderly people are on indigestion tablets that lower the amount of stomach acid available. This means that a vitamin B12 deficiency is potentially likely to occur.

Good sources of vitamin B are:

- Wheat germ
- Wholemeal bread
- Yeast extract, Marmite, for example
- Nuts and seeds
- Liver and kidney

Vitamin B12 is found in animal protein sources only. Vegetarians will have to supplement this vitamin as it cannot be obtained from plant sources. Supplements of B12 are inevitably made from animal sources.

The fat soluble vitamins

Dietary links to Alzheimer's Disease were discovered in 1999 and were more recently updated. The main findings were that excessive dietary fat and energy were high risk factors for Alzheimer's disease. However, there are various forms of fat and some reduce the risk for the dementias. This particular study also found significantly reduced risk factors for those eating fish and cereals. The latter findings have been supported in various epidemiological studies. We shall look at all these findings later.

There are four fat soluble vitamins. These are the vitamins ADEK. Most people are aware of vitamin A and D and know that vitamin D is referred to as the 'sunshine vitamin.' This is because it can be made by the action of the sun's rays on the skin. Vitamin D will be looked at in more detail under the chapter entitled Sunlight and Exercise.

All fat soluble vitamins need to be taken with a little fat in the diet in order to be absorbed. This needs to be emphasised. Vitamin D that is bought off the shelves of supermarkets are often in 'hard' tablet form. If they are swallowed without the presence of a small amount of fat, then the vitamin cannot be absorbed.

Vitamin C and vitamin E work together in the brain. Vitamin E is the most abundant fat soluble antioxidant in the body, as such it is vital for keeping the fatty tissue in the brain healthy. Vitamin C neutralises toxic oxidants but it goes further than this; it helps recycle the vitamin E residue and reactivates it.

Of course, the sooner that adequate amounts of vitamin C and vitamin E are included in the diet the sooner any preclinical damage can be turned around.

It is not surprising that smokers have a higher risk for dementia since every cigarette uses up approximately 30mg of vitamin C. The recommended daily allowance is 30mg so it can be seen that smokers use up every scrap of the recommended vitamin C intake in one cigarette. Once this is used up, then free radicals are generated galore. This will, of course, impact on the body's ability to recycle and reactivate vitamin E. It is not surprising that smokers have a much higher risk of dementia than non-smokers.

Of course, some other jobs that may increase the risk include those working with pesticides, chemicals of any sort, those working where the air is polluted. Lorry drivers constantly travelling up and down the motorways, are just some examples of individuals working in polluted environments.

Those people with digestive issues such as Crohn's disease, where absorption of food is compromised, will also need to pay special attention to their intake of the antioxidant vitamins and minerals which are known to impact the brain positively.

Vitamin E is found in wheat germ, nuts, seeds and dark green leafy vegetable. If it is added to food you will see the word tocopherol somewhere in the ingredients list.

The recommended dietary allowance is 400 mg daily.

Other vital antioxidants

There are four other antioxidants that play a vital role in the health of the brain. These are:

- Zinc
- Selenium
- Co-enzyme Q10
- Turmeric

Zinc

In the apparently healthy elderly, deficiencies of zinc and vitamin C are ranked as the first and second major cause of micronutrient deficiencies and these deficiencies are also considered to be risk factors for herpes zoster and post herpetic neuralgia as well as Alzheimer's disease. All of these conditions are rife in the elderly population.

Zinc can be depleted by excessive intake of copper, so if you have a diet that is excessively high in copper then you may need to make some changes and include more zinc or reduce the intake of copper containing foods.

Zinc is a great antiviral and will be required to deal with any inflammation cause by a virus. A study of Taiwanese patients with post herpetic neuralgia found that they were deficient in zinc. Therefore, if a person has shingles and/or post herpetic neuralgia then this poses the question whether generalised subclinical inflammation – also a characteristic of dementia - is occurring.

As zinc is a trace element, it is required in very small amounts in our body. In spite of this it has a number of important roles that impact on the health of the brain. For example, zinc is required to activate an immune cell called a T lymphocyte. These T cells are important because they

- help regulate immune responses
- attack infected or cancerous cells

Studies[2] have shown that when bacteria is injected into murine brains then beta amyloid was formed as a defence. When the plaques were looked at each one had a single bacterium in it.

This suggests that it is an infection that is the underlying cause of Alzheimer's disease. The beta amyloid plaques are trapping any microbes that are crossing the blood brain barrier. If they can't be carried away quickly enough then their build up causes the tangles that are characteristic of Alzheimer's disease. As zinc increases immune cells that attack infected cells, then this may reduce the need for the synthesis of beta amyloid as a defensive measure against microbes that have crossed the blood brain barrier.

The normal recommended dietary allowance of zinc is:

- 11mg for men
- 8mg for women

---

[2] https://www.newscientist.com/article/2090221-alzheimers-may-be-caused-by-brains-sticky-defence-against-bugs/

Good sources of zinc include:

- Meat
- Shellfish
- Beans, chickpeas, lentils and other legumes
- Eggs
- Whole grains
- Nuts
- Dairy
- seeds

Selenium

Selenium is an essential trace element that is an excellent antioxidant. Many people are deficient in selenium. Our impoverished soil is selenium deficient

---

1. [3] Vural H, Demirin H, Kara Y, Eren I, Delibas N. Alterations of Plasmamagnesium, Copper, Zinc, Iron and Selenium Concentrations and Some Related Erythrocyte Antioxidant Enzyme Activities in Patients with Alzheimer's Disease. JTrace Elem Med Biol. 2010 Jul;24(3):169–73. doi: 10.1016/j.jtemb.2010.02.002

which means that our food will also be deficient in this mineral.

Some studies[3] have shown that there is a significant reduction in levels of selenium in those with Alzheimer's disease. Other studies do not show such differences. We cannot discount the role of selenium as a protective factor against Alzheimer's disease since there is unlikely to be just one causative factor in the build-up of beta amyloid protein. It is likely that there are a number of causative factors and that each individual will have their own contributory factors. Changing just one of these factors may well change the whole progression and outcome of the disease.

Good food sources of selenium are:

- Brewer's yeast
- Garlic
- Liver
- Eggs
- mushrooms

Animal sources of selenium are much higher than those from plants. It is interesting to note that deficiencies of selenium can result in premature ageing and nerve disorders. Two brazil nuts can supply the daily recommended amount but, as selenium is toxic, it is advised that the recommended daily allowance of 200 micrograms is not exceeded.

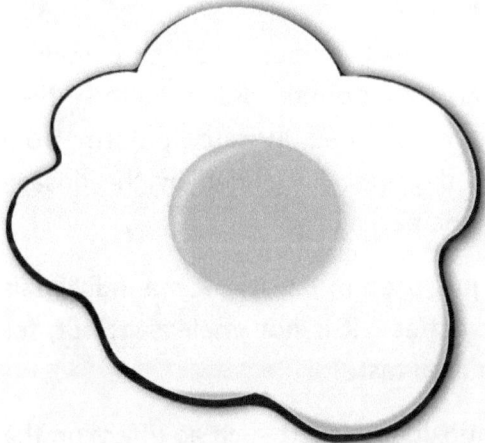

Eggs are a good source of selenium.

Turmeric (curcumin)

Turmeric – the yellow spice that is used in curries – contains a substance known as curcumin. Curcumin has anti-inflammatory properties This substance reduces oxidised LDL cholesterol and protects artery walls from the effects of homocysteine. Homocysteine is an amino acid by product which can damage blood vessel walls. Numerous studies have shown that people in countries - where turmeric/curcumin is eaten on a regular basis - suffer less dementia. However, curcumin has another valuable property – that of being able to break down amyloid beta protein ready for removal to the blood stream.

There are only small amounts of curcumin in turmeric. If larger amounts are required, then curcumin can be obtained in capsule form from most health food stores. Be guided by the dosage instructions on the packaging.

Turmeric isn't just used in curries. Some individuals make turmeric coffee. It is not unpleasant but, for me, it is an acquired taste!

Why should antioxidants exert such an effect on the brain? Well. antioxidants help bring oxygen to the brain as well as reducing the likelihood of damaging oxidation.

Studies have shown that individuals who have elevated levels of vitamin E, C and A in their diets score better in memory tests.

Table showing food sources of antioxidants

Antioxidant	Sources
Anthocyanins	Grapes, berries, aubergine
Sulphur compounds	Onions, leeks and garlic
Beta carotene	Carrots, pumpkin, mangoes, apricots, spinach and parsley
Catechins	Tea and red wine
Copper	Seafood, milk, nuts, meat, cocoa and dark chocolate
Cryptoxanthin	Mangoes, pumpkin, red pepper
Flavonoids	Tea, red wine, onion, apple, citrus fruit
Indoles	Cruciferous vegetables such as cabbage and cauliflower
Isoflavonoids	Lentils, peas, milk, tofu, soya products
Lignans	Bran, whole grains, vegetables, seeds such as linseed
Lutein	Leafy greens such as kale, chard and spinach
Lycopene	Tomatoes, pink grapefruit, watermelon
Manganese	Lean meat, nuts, milk, seafood
Polyphenols	Aromatic herbs such as

	thyme and oregano
Selenium	Brazil nuts (not more than two daily) seafood, whole grains organ meats
Antioxidant	Food source
Vitamin C	Fresh fruit and vegetables
Vitamin E	Vegetable oils and whole grains. However, many vegetable oils create inflammation and are better avoided altogether. Olive oil, however, is a mono-saturated oil and is not proinflammatory. This can be used freely. Keep it stored in the fridge in darkness
Zinc	Nuts, milk, seafood and lean meat

Co-enzyme Q10

Co-enzyme Q10 is a vitamin like substance that is generally found in organ meats and sea food. It is essential for neuromuscular function and respiration of cells that is undertaken by mitochondria.

The poor functioning of mitochondria is associated with the early stages of dementia. Beta amyloid appears to be toxic to mitochondria.

CoQ10 protects and helps boost mitochondrial energy production.

Recent studies[4] have shown that when neuronal cells are treated with an CoQ10 analogue then they are protected from oligomeric amyloid beta protein. This is the main form found in the pathology of Alzheimer's disease.

CoQ10 by neutralising free radicals, increases a substance called NF-kB which I shall refer to as Kappa B. Kappa B helps prevent the release of substances that promote inflammation. This is a useful protective factor for most inflammatory diseases including the dementias.

Co-enzyme Q10 becomes depleted with age, illness and statin use and supplements may be necessary. It is easily obtainable in capsule form from any health food store.

Good sources of Coenzyme Q10 are:

- Mackerel
- Seafood of any sort
- Liver
- Kidneys
- Heart

---

[4] https://mitochondrialdiseasenews.com/2018/01/29

- Other meats have lesser - but still valuable - quantities

When younger, the majority of CoQ10 is synthesised internally from two amino acids and another substance.

- Tyrosine (amino acid)
- Phenylananine (amino acid)
- Mevalonic acid

Ageing decreases production so dietary intake is an important consideration in later life.

Good sources of tyrosine - which is eventually converted to phenylalanine - are:

- Turkey and chicken
- Fish
- Milk and other dairy products
- Peanuts, almonds pumpkin and sesame seeds
- Lima beans
- Bananas
- Soy products

Although we have looked at antioxidants that help reduce inflammation, we did begin this book by stating that some foods did generate free radicals that cause inflammation. A diet full of antioxidants does contribute to the slowing of the development of Alzheimer's Disease by modulating oxidative stress and inflammation. The dementias may also arise from the production of series 2 prostaglandins (from arachidonic acid) which we shall look at in more detail later. Arachidonic acid also helps to promote colon cancer).[5]

By far the biggest culprit is sugar. There are a number of studies that show that when blood sugar spikes it produces an inflammatory response in the linings of arteries. This inflammatory response is characteristic of vascular dementia.

The second biggest contributor to inflammation are the pro-inflammatory omega 6 oils. It is to these that we will now turn our attention.

---

[5] Fan YY et al Carcinogenesis 2014

The Good, the Bad and the Ugly about Fats, Oils and anti-cholinergic medications

Ask most older people about saturated fats and they will be able to name a string of them at once. They were brought up on them. They formed part of the diet during the war and immediate post war years. They provided much needed calories and fat soluble vitamins – the latter of which are often lacking in our diet.

Saturated fats are those fats which are solid at room temperature – butter, lard, dripping, meat and coconut oil are examples of saturated fat.

Saturated fats are another substance which have become demonised even though studies show that they raise HDL – the lipoprotein that is labelled as 'good cholesterol.

Saturated fat also changes the pattern of LDL, increasing the subgroup of LDL which transports much needed substances for cell growth and repair. Studies have shown that saturated fat is associated with less coronary atherosclerosis than it if it is replaced by other food groups. When saturated fat is replaced with carbohydrate, for example, then the progression of atherosclerosis is greater. Further, when saturated fats are replaced with unsaturated fats, the progression of atherosclerosis also increases.

Lard could be considered a superfood. It is the second richest source of Vitamin D and is rich in cholesterol. It does not contain trans-fat – the real culprit behind heart disease and a major contributor to brain degeneration. It contains 60% monounsaturated fat which is associated with a decreased risk of heart disease. Monounsaturated fats also decrease inflammation. This is one of our prime tasks in the fight against neurodegeneration.

Saturated fat has many advantages over other fats for cooking. It is far more stable and so is less likely to be damaged when heated than, for example, oils such as olive oil or rape seed oil. This means it hardly generates free radicals that are implicated in the dementias.

Poly- unsaturated fatty acids.

 A further group of fats - The poly unsaturated fats - are the omega 6's and the omega 3's - docosahexaenoic acid (DHA) and eicosapentoic acid (EPA). These are liquid at room temperature.

The polyunsaturated fatty acid found in omega six oils is called linoleic acid. It is derived from vegetable oils and it is a major player in fuelling inflammatory processes. Neurodegeneration and inflammation go hand in hand.

Our diet is full of omega 6 without us realising it. These vegetable oils are added to just about every food on the market. It is hidden in biscuits and cakes, added to tinned soups etc., it is now used for cooking fish and chips, when dripping was once used.

Most of the population are not aware of how much ubiquitous pro-inflammatory oil they are ingesting. When it comes to saturated fat and omega 6, it cannot be repeated enough that it is the latter that creates inflammation. Studies show that it is the balance between omega 6 and omega three which impacts far more on health than any concerns we may erroneously have about saturated fat. We should be eating far more omega 3 in our diet than we currently are and the amount of omega 6's should be limited significantly, if they have to be used.

Arachidonic acid is a polyunsaturated omega-6 fatty acid. It is found in the membranes of the body's cells and is particularly abundant in the brain, muscles and liver. It is a key inflammatory intermediate and can act as a vasodilator. This means it can widen blood vessels.

Arachidonic acid has many beneficial roles in the body. It will not cause inflammation unless tiny particles, called electrons, try and disrupt the stability of other electrons found in the fat that forms part of the cell membranes.

Arachidonic acid can be metabolised to both anti-inflammatory and proinflammatory eicanosoids. Eicanosoids are the end product of a series of metabolic processes. It is quite likely that if you suffer from joint pain, bronchoconstriction, microvascular permeability and lymphoedema that arachidonic acid has been converted to a pro-inflammatory compound.

There are numerous studies that show that arachidonic acid is implicated in Alzheimer's disease. Arachidonic acid activates enzymes called kinases. These kinases appear to increase tau phosphorylation levels. This just means that more phosphate is added to the tau protein that is characteristic of Alzheimer's disease.

Free arachidonic acid can be converted to substances that contribute to the occurrence and progression of neuroinflammation.[6] Studies have shown that arachidonic acid is involved in bringing about the beta amyloid plaques in mouse models.

Essential fatty acids (EFA's) are vital for the health of the brain and regulate many of the processes that have been pathologically altered in Alzheimer's disease. These processes resulted in learning, memory and behavioural impairments in the mouse models.

---

[6] https://www.jneurology.com/articles/arachidonic-acid-in-alzheimers-disease.html

While some nutrients can be made within the body, EFA's cannot. They have to be taken in through diet on a daily basis.

Omega 3 oils contain alpha linoleic acid. Alpha linoleic acid is found in walnuts and flaxseeds. It is an essential fatty acid. It is anti-inflammatory and good for reducing inflammation in arteries.

Two long chain omega three fatty acids that you should become familiar with are

- Eicosapentenoic acid (EPA) and
- Docosahexaenoic acid (DHA)

As EPA and DHA can compete with arachidonic acid for the synthesis of eicosanoids then it is to our advantage that we take in more of these - than arachidonic acid - as they tip the balance towards less inflammatory activity.

There should be about six times the amount of omega 3's ingested to the omega 6's. The reality is that it is the other way around. We are eating far too many vegetable oils containing the pro-inflammatory omega 6 fatty acids. In other words, we are providing the fuel for a state of chronic inflammation including neurodegeneration.

The Victorians suffered very little heart disease in spite of their high saturated fat diet which was full of lard, dripping, eggs and butter. In fact, heart disease wasn't considered important enough to study at medical school in those times, since there was so little of it. Dementia is also a new disease on the block. We shall look at the reasons and evidence for this later.

Eventually these important saturated fats were replaced with the 'healthier' substitutes of.

- Omega 6 vegetable oils
- margarine

Crisco was one of the first new fats to be introduced to the unsuspecting public. It was promoted as making flakier pastry. It was full of trans fats. Trans fats are toxic to the human body.

Other important fats vital for brain and eye health are eggs.

Eggs were demonised as being full of 'bad' cholesterol. People were frightened to eat one of the most nutritionally and complete foods to be found. The 'Go to work on an egg' was replaced by messages that eggs contained salmonella and should be avoided. The junior minister – Edwina Currie – eventually had to resign from her post after the British Egg Industry Council called her remarks 'factually incorrect and highly irresponsible' saying that the risk of being infected with salmonella was less than 200 million to one.

Since saturated fats were replaced with 'healthier' substitutes, heart disease and neurodegenerative disease have increased markedly. Further, the introduction of cholesterol lowering drugs – which occurred more or less at the same time as these dietary changes - provide cogent explanations for the increase in chronic diseases.

Dr Weil M.D. in his book Healthy Aging observed that during the plenary presentations of the 11th Anti-Aging Conference and Exposition that it was mooted that chronic inflammation was a common root of neuro-degenerative disorders including Alzheimer disease, Parkinson's disease and Amyotrophic Sclerosis. It was emphasised that dietary modifications were a treatment strategy – a view point which I also hold. However, it is unlikely to be promoted as a treatment strategy. It does not hold any profit for the pharmaceutical companies.

Monounsaturated fats help promote a healthy blood flow to the brain. They help to produce and release acetylcholine which is essential for learning and memory; the loss of acetylcholine will result in memory problems often associated with Alzheimer's disease. It seems apt to include a small section on anti-cholinergic drugs here although this book is primarily about diet.

Anti-cholinergic drugs

Anti-cholinergic drugs oppose the action of the neurotransmitter acetylcholine. They inhibit the transmission of parasympathetic nerve impulses and reduce spasms of smooth muscles. They also inhibit learning and the formation of memories. Studies show that individuals who have taken anti-cholinergics have a significant degree of cognitive impairment. Further, there were physical differences in the brains of participants in the study, that were not found in individuals who had not taken anti-cholinergics. Those who had taken anti-cholinergics were found to have pathological changes in their brain tissue that was characteristic of Alzheimer's disease.

Are anti-cholinergics popular medicine? Yes! They are found in many over the counter medications especially in anti-allergy medications that are routinely taken by many.

Common anti-cholinergics are:
- Benadryl
- Medications taken by individual's with Parkinson's disease.
- Combivent for asthma
- Chlorpheniramine (Actifed Allergy for congestion relief)
- Tylenol PM

31

- Nortriptyline
- Amitriptyline
- Phenergan
- Ditropan

Studies have shown that these anti-cholinergic medications do not have to be taken for long periods of time to raise the risk for the pathological changes leading to a diagnosis of Alzheimer's disease. Sporadic and limited use also increase the risk.

Most people will have taken one or more of these medications during their lifetime. It is no wonder, given the introduction of these drugs – and the ease with which they can be obtained – that dementia is so prevalent in society.

Conclusion

At the end of this long chapter on inflammation, free radicals and antioxidants, these important points have been raised.

- *Saturated fat needs to replace vegetable oils such as rape seed, canola, sunflower oil. Saturated fats are stable fats and do not increase the potential for inflammation. They do not cause atherosclerotic plaques.*

- *A suitable oil that can also be used is olive oil which is a monounsaturated fatty acid. This does not cause inflammation.*
- *Avoid processed foods that have few antioxidants and may contain harmful poly-unsaturated omega 6's.*
- *Eat foods containing zinc, turmeric, selenium and coenzymeQ10 regularly.*
- *Do not be fearful of eating saturated fats such as dripping, butter and lard. They contain vital fat soluble vitamins that are necessary for brain health. In addition, they are a good source of vitamin D that helps regulate inflammatory processes. Vitamin D also produces an anti-microbial called cathelicidin that tackles a number of infective agents.*
- *Avoid anti-cholinergic medication.*

Neurotransmitters: the messenger boys

Neurotransmitters are the messenger boys in the brain. They are manufactured from amino acids and send messages from cell to cell.

Acetylcholine is a critical neurotransmitter for memory. It helps us to retain any memories that are formed. There is a link between low levels of acetylcholine in the hippocampus and neocortex areas of the brain and Alzheimer's disease.

Specifically, two substances are crucial for the manufacture of acetylcholine and these are:

- Glycine
- Choline

Glycine – the smallest amino acid – is a non-essential amino acid. By implication, it is thought that all our requirements are manufactured in the body. However, a deficiency is implicated in many disease states. Glycine infusion has been found to prevent microglial activation which is implicated in the progression of some neurodegenerative disorders. Microglia are a type of immune system cell. When they are present in greater numbers it shows disease progression.

Increasing glycine intake has also been found to reverse type 2 diabetes   Type 2 diabetes is a risk factor for dementia. Other studies have also shown that autistic spectrum disorder is a manifestation of glycine deficiency. It occurs as a result of the consumption of a typical diet that is high in essential amino acids but lacking in glycine.

Where is this amazing glycine to be found. In the 1940's and 1950's glycine would be found in abundance in most people's diets. Nowadays, rarely so. Glycine is found in properly made bone broth, fish head soup, pork crackling, organ meats, proper home-made ox tail soup and chicken skin, among others. In fact, most of the foods that we do not eat nowadays!

Any food that contain gelatine will also contain glycine. There are not many vegetarian sources that contain large enough amounts of glycine but they include beans and spinach.   Jelly is also a good source as are wine gums. Many of the confectionary products available in the immediate post war years were based on gelatine and its amazing chewy texture. Not many people knew it was a protein product with medicinal value.

Powdered gelatine can be purchased at most health food stores and online. It is flavourless and can be sprinkled over food although it has a slightly gritty texture. Alternatively, it can be bloomed in a little water before being added to stock or soup. Some people bloom gelatine and add it to coffee. It is a matter of personal preference.

Some of glycine's other amazing properties centre on its inhibitory properties. It thus helps to reduce pain, aids sleep and lessens anxiety. Thus, it is a vital substance to help control the symptoms found in the dementias.

The steps that glycine must go through before forming acetylcholine are: glycine-serine-taurine ADD thyroxine + choline ⟹ acetylcholine.

Choline

Choline is an essential nutrient that is naturally present in some foods. It is a source of methyl groups. Methyl groups are required to complete metabolic steps. Choline's importance becomes more urgent when folate levels are low. Folate is the main methyl donor for metabolic pathways. When it is not available in sufficient amounts them choline becomes the primary source.

Choline is required to synthesise phosphatidylcholine which is required for the structural integrity of cell membranes. Although individual's can make some in the body, this is not generally enough for the body's needs.

Choline is stored in the liver and phosphorylated when required to make cell membranes. Requirements for choline are influenced by the amount of available methionine, betaine and folate in the diet.

Good sources are:

- Meat
- Poultry
- Fish
- Dairy products
- Eggs
- Cruciferous vegetables
- Beans
- Nuts and seeds
- Whole grains

Adequate intakes are deemed to be:

Male: 550mg/daily

Female 425mg/daily

Choline is currently not added to parenteral nutrition.

Studies have found that individuals with Alzheimer's Disease have lower levels of the enzyme that converts choline into acetylcholine.

For those that like the challenge of chemistry:

Acetylcholine is synthesised from acetyl coenzyme A and choline by the enzyme choline acetyltransferase in the nervous system. There are some inhibitors of acetylcholinesterase that are not reversible. They are used in insecticides and chemical warfare agents.

It is reasonable to assume that those who have come into contact with these type of substances may have lower levels of this enzyme and have a reduced conversion of choline into acetylcholine. If an individual has worked with insecticides either in paid work or at home or further, been subject to chemical warfare agents then these are risk factors for dementia.

Of course, it is clear that a diet must contain sufficient choline to be converted into acetylcholine if any potential increase in memory problems due to this are to be avoided.

We could also try and retain the acetylcholine that is available for a little longer. This would involve inhibiting the enzyme responsible for the breakdown of acetylcholine, that is the enzyme cholinesterase. We shall consider this in more detail in the chapter entitled DMSO.

Table of foods containing good sources of choline

Beef liver – fried 3 ounces	356mg
egg	147mg
beef	117mg
Soybean ½ cup	107mg
Chicken breast cooked	72 mg
Ground beef- three ounces	71mg
Shitake mushrooms sliced ½ cup	58mg
potatoes	57mg

Foods containing cholesterol are the main forms of dietary choline. As such, those on statins, have an increased risk for neurodegeneration and associated dementia. This risk factor has been born out in numerous studies.

Why is Alzheimer's a new disease and what can be done about it?

Fish oil has been found to elevate a protein that prevents the formation of amyloid beta protein that is found in the brains of those with Alzheimer's disease. Researchers found that the omega-3 fatty acid docosahexanoic acid that is found in fish oil, increases a substance known as LR11. LR11 helps to destroy the plaques found in the disease. It has been found that those individuals with reduced levels of DHA either have Alzheimer's disease or are at high risk of being diagnosed with it.

As I have already discussed, the imbalance of poly unsaturated fatty acids omega 3's and omega's 6's has a major negative impact on our health including the health of the brain.

When we look at the incidence of Alzheimer's disease we find that it is a fairly 'new' disease. Studies[7] have shown that it was very rare or did not exist prior to 1900. However, it did develop a rapidly increasing prevalence after about 1950 – more or less as the inflammatory vegetable oils were introduced as the new health food.

There is further evidence that supports the introduction of inflammatory oils as a causative factor for Alzheimer's disease'

---

[7]

https://www.frontiersin.org/articles/10.3389/fnagi.2014.00092/full

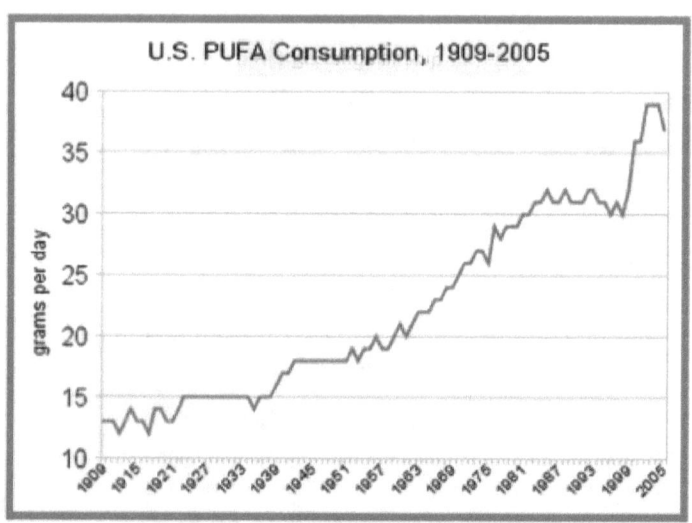

Poly-unsaturated Fatty Acid Consumption

8

Waldeman and Lamb's book Dying for a Hamburger examined this new disease. They highlighted that Osler, who edited a text book of all known diseases in the late 1800s did not identify a condition like Alzheimer's disease. This is not because Osler could not identify diseases of the brain. Apparently he devoted one whole volume to neurological conditions. It just appears that Alzheimer's disease did not exist at the time and therefore he could not include it.

---

[8] https://medium.com/@drjasonfung/the-shocking-origin-of-vegetable-oil-garbage-1c2ce14ae513

Boyd, another author of textbooks of pathology, during the late 1800's did not identify - nor describe - any amyloid plaques or neurofibrillary tangles in his numerous autopsies.   This is further evidence that Alzheimer's disease did not exist at that time.

Could it be that those in the late 1800's did not live long enough to develop Alzheimer's commonly seen as a disease of old age? Well, no!   The age of onset of dementia is 60 years of age and there were still a few million people living beyond that age without any signs of dementia.

Environmental Copper

Environmental copper is a substance that is found widely in our home and working environments. It is a metal that is released into the environment by human activity as well as natural sources. Decaying vegetation, sea spray, forest fires, dust release copper. Plumbers and builders, among others, use copper in the course of their working day. It is found in phosphate fertiliser production, landfill, waste disposal sites and in homes where there is copper piping.

Studies have shown that copper reduces the rate of clearance of amyloid beta from brain to blood. We have already discussed that it is the slow clearance of beta amyloid from the brain that is implicated in the pathology of Alzheimer's disease.

The 'antidote' to too much copper is zinc. Zinc and copper compete for absorption in the gut. Zinc has also been found to protect against reactive oxygen species (ROS) by binding to amyloid beta protein. By binding to amyloid beta protein in the place of copper there is a decrease of Reactive Oxygen Species created. Further, zinc is able to reduce the toxic effect of amyloid beta protein by changing these proteins into less harmful shapes. As we have already seen, Zinc has other useful properties when it comes to addressing some of the sub clinical processes that may lead to a diagnosis of dementia. It also now appears to be able to reduce the risk produced by environmental (unbound) copper.

Coffee

Coffee has been proven to reverse the memory impairment in animal models of dementia. There may be a number of reasons for this. Coffee is a powerful antioxidant, quenching free radicals that contribute to inflammation.

A study[9] argued that the human body is in a constant battle to keep from aging. Research[10] suggests that free

---

[9] https://www.ncbi.nlm.nih.gov/pmc/articles/PMC3249911/

[10] Ashok BT, Ali R. The aging paradox: Free radical theory of aging. Exp Gerontol. 1999; 34:293–303.

radical damage to cells leads to the pathological changes associated with ageing.

Studies[11] have shown that coffee drinkers are less likely to get ALS, Parkinson's disease and Alzheimer's disease. These are all diseases of advancing age. In a study[3] of elderly mice with Alzheimer's disease, for example, caffeine was found to reverse cognitive impairment as well as lowering brain amyloid-beta levels.

In an animal model of ALS, coffee was found to increase antioxidant enzyme capacity in the brain of male G39A mice, improving motor performance.

A caffeine derivative, known as LM11A-24 appears to protect degenerating motor neurons.[12]

This is all well and good; coffee, whether it is decaffeinated, or not, has been found to slow down the progression of neurodegeneration.

Coffee contains a number of important antioxidants as well as vitamin B3. Niacin is added to – and found in- a great many foods so it is less likely that this is the important nutrient that slows the progression of brain degeneration.

Science Direct[13] states that:

---

[11] https://academic.oup.com/aje/article/174/9/1002/168671
[12] https://www.ncbi.nlm.nih.gov/pubmed/17004921
[13]

Coffee beans are a rich source of biologically active compounds such as caffeine, chlorogenic acids, nicotinic acid, trigonelline, cafestol, and kahweol, which have significant potential as antioxidants.

It is worth exploring these antioxidants a little further.

Chlorogenic acids

These have a wide array of benefits including having an anti-inflammatory effect in the brain.

Trigonelline –

This substance has many potential benefits.[14] It is neuroprotective, anti-migraine and reduces neuron excitability.

Cafestol and kahweol

Both of these substances tend to impact positively on the liver lowering inflammation in this organ. There are studies[15] that link liver and gut activity with Alzheimer's disease. The brain is intricately connected to all other organs.

---

https://www.sciencedirect.com/science/article/pii/B97801240473 89000039

[14] https://www.researchgate.net/publication/225288518_Trigonellin e_A_Plant_Alkaloid_with_Therapeutic_Potential_for_Diabetes_and _Central_Nervous_System_Disease

[15] https://www.alzheimersresearchuk.org/new-findings-link-activity-gut-liver-alzheimers-risk/

Whole wheat grains have powerful antioxidant activity

A study[16] showed that wheat, one of the most important grains in the world, is not only a source of basic nutrients, such as carbohydrates, proteins, and vitamins, but also a source of antioxidants, such as flavonoids and phenolic acids. It was reported that the antioxidant activity of whole grain including whole wheat bread ranged from 1303 to 2479 µmol trolox *** equivalent (TE) per 100 g, whereas the average values of 24 types of fruit and 22 types of vegetables were 2200 and 1200 µmol TE per 100 g, respectively. These results indicated that whole grains have pronounced antioxidant activities that should not be overlooked.

When was white bread introduced into the UK? This occurred around the 1950's at the same time that vegetable oils took off. One product – white bread - lacked the antioxidant properties of wholegrain loaves and the other – the pro inflammatory oils - replaced our saturated fats full of brain healthy vitamins and replaced it with a bottle full of inflammation!

16

https://www.sciencedirect.com/science/article/pii/S221451411500
0471
***A trolox is basically the strength of antioxidant activity

Is there anything else we can learn about the dementias from our erroneously 'new and improved' diet? As vegetable oils (omega 6's) increase inflammation within arteries, they are also a risk factor for heart disease. In fact, studies[17] show that 30% of people with Alzheimer's disease also have heart disease and 29% also have diabetes.

There are only limited sources of omega 3 fatty acid and these are:

- Oily fish such as mackerel, salmon, fresh tuna, pilchard
- Eggs (if the hens have been fed with products containing omega 3)
- Algae (the vegetarian form of DHA omega 3 is made from this source.)

From these fairly limited sources, it is unlikely that we are ingesting enough omega 3's while it is practically impossible to avoid the omega 6's. If we are not prepared to make oily fish a part of our daily diet, then we need to supplement with DHA. Until the ratio of omega 3 fatty acids and omega 6 fatty acids is in the ratio of 6:1 then low grade systemic inflammation will occur

---

[17] https://www.alzheimers.net/resources/alzheimers-statistics/

Further evidence of the anti-inflammatory effects of omega three fatty acids comes from a study by Professor Swank who looked at the diets of mountain dwelling and sea dwelling populations in relation to the incidence of multiple sclerosis found in those populations.

The mountain dwellers ate mainly meat and those by the sea, fish. There were diagnosed cases of multiple sclerosis in the mountain dwellers. Those populations of sea dwellers were not diagnosed with multiple sclerosis. Of course, it could be argued that it was not the presence of omega three oils that had a protective effect. Fish, has an amino acid, taurine, that has many beneficial effects and is associated with longevity. Nevertheless, there are many supportive studies for the benefits of docosahexanoic acid for those with neurodegeneration.

What do we conclude from the evidence that has been gathered so far? We can reasonably assume that Alzheimer's disease and vascular dementia are diseases of civilisation. Both these dementias are barely heard of in undeveloped countries. Japan is the only developed country that appears to have very low rates of dementia.

When we look at the diet of the Japanese it is full of zinc and DHA and both these nutrients are known to positively impact on the brain. Their diet is high in grains and vegetables. Fish is often eaten raw thereby retaining he antioxidants that are also to be found in fish.

The diet of the long-lived Okinawan people has not been influenced by western culture as much as other parts of Japan. This may explain why they are a community of people who often reach ages of over one hundred years. However, throughout Japan, Alzheimer is a little known disease.

Protective factors for Alzheimer's Disease

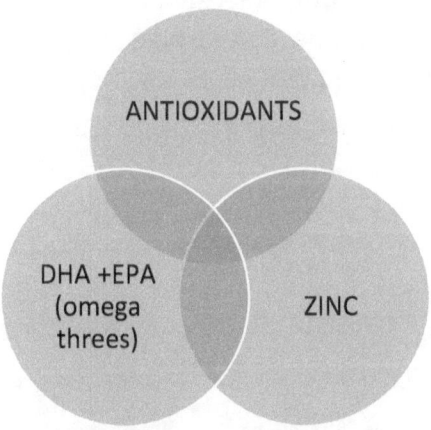

Sleep and beta amyloid

Although this book is about dietary factors that may prevent subclinical Alzheimer's dementia - or help to reduce the rate of progression once a diagnosis has been made - it would be remiss of me not to highlight the importance of good quality sleep in the battle against dementia.

Chronic sleep disorders are associated with Alzheimer's disease. It is thought that during sleep the brain clears out amyloid beta plaques.

Insomnia is a complex problem that may be caused by a number of reasons including stress, anxiety, looking at screens which prevents the production of melatonin, the sleep hormone.

For a more comprehensive look at sleep disorders and how they can be overcome the book [18]Sleep, Perchance to Dream, by Lynne D M Noble, covers most of the common sleep problems.

A Triad of Risk Factors in the dementias

---

[18] https://www.amazon.co.uk/dp/1791728332

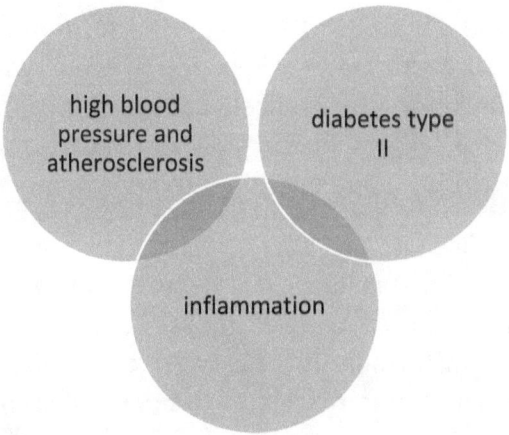

The interconnectedness of high blood pressure and atherosclerosis, diabetes type II and inflammation are well established. They have been identified as significant risk factors for vascular dementia.

If we take diabetes type II we can see how it is associated with high blood pressure and atherosclerosis.

The high blood sugar levels found in diabetes type II lay down sticky plaque in the lining of the arteries. As the arteries narrow, the heart has to pump harder to push the blood through narrowed arteries raising blood pressure. If any of the plaque, lining the arteries, breaks off it may travel to the brain and lodge in the smaller vessels cutting off the blood supply. When the brain is deprived of oxygen and nutrients then vascular dementia occurs.

Low grade chronic Inflammation contributes to our triad of risk factors so antioxidants are one weapon in this battle. What are the likely causes of inflammation? Sugar is the biggest factor, poly unsaturated omega 6 oils are a close second and, then there is homocysteine.

Homocysteine is an amino acid that should be a temporary by product in a cycle known as the methionine cycle. However, in order that homocysteine can be transformed into a less toxic substance, it requires a number of the B complex vitamins to be available. If these are in short supply, then homocysteine deposits itself in the lining of arteries and 'roughs' them up. Cells of the immune system that respond to inflammation gather at these sites narrowing the diameter of blood vessels.

It has been argued that cholesterol is also responsible for atherosclerosis since it is sometimes found in arteries. However, there are reasons why this is unlikely to be the case. Cholesterol is required to maintain the integrity of all cell membranes. It is the LDL – the supposedly 'bad' cholesterol that is carried to sites of injury. However, it does this in order to repair damage to cells. Cholesterol also helps to reduce infection. There are numerous studies that show that those with higher cholesterol levels are less likely to die from infection. Studies have also implicated bacterial infections in the genesis and progression of Alzheimer's disease. This may also be true of vascular dementia. Further, there are a number of studies that associate high LDL levels with better cognition. Those individuals with high LDL levels appear to have better memories in older age.

How do you increase the B complex in your diet especially vitamin B3, B6 and folic acid? Wholegrains, nut, seeds, yeast and fortified cereals are good sources of the B complex as well as excellent sources of antioxidants. Vitamin B supplements can also be found very cheaply at supermarkets and generally are composed of the full range of B complex.

Vitamin B complex is a water soluble vitamin and is easily destroyed or leached into water during cooking processes. Therefore, light cooking using a minimum amount of water is recommended.

Protective factors in vascular dementia

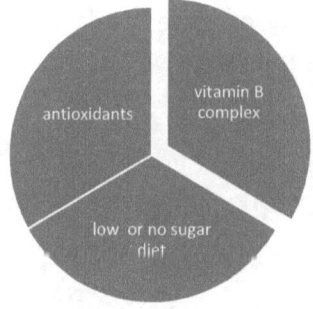

Further risk factors for vascular dementia

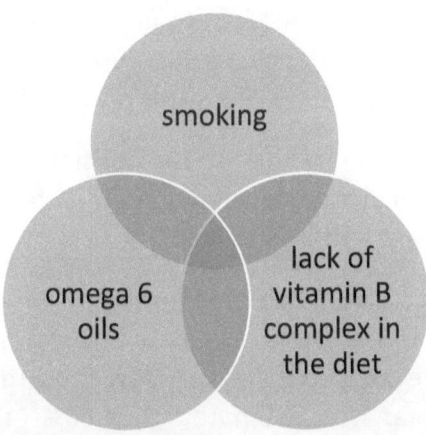

- Smoking reduces vitamin C which has a powerful anti-inflammatory action.
- Omega 6 oils are inflammatory in nature.
- Vitamin B prevents plaque from sticking to the inner linings of arteries and setting up an inflammatory action.

The importance of exercise and sunlight

Exercise is essential in the fight against dementia. Exercise promotes circulation of the blood which carries life giving nutrients and oxygen to where they are required. As most exercise is undertaken outside then there is also the chance to soak up vitamin D that is made from the action of the sun's rays on the skin.

Research does show that those deficient in vitamin D are twice as likely to develop dementia than those who aren't deficient in this vitamin.

Vitamin D is clearly important for the health of the brain as vitamin D receptors are found throughout neural tissue. However, there are very few foods that contain vitamin D and it is estimated that 80% of the world population are vitamin D deficient.

There are also many groups of people who are at particular risk of vitamin D deficiency:

Those people who are particularly likely to be at risk of a vitamin D deficiency.

Older People — because:

Skin gets thinner as you get older. This makes it harder to make Vitamin D when it is exposed to sunlight.

- Older people tend to eat less and also tend to spend more time indoors – both these will reduce the amount of vitamin D someone has in their system.

People with Darker Skin because:

- The melanin in their skin helps protect them from the sun's ultra violet rays which reduces the body's ability to make this vitamin from the sun.

People with medical conditions that reduce fat absorption and those on low fat diets because:

- Vitamin D is fat soluble and needs a properly functioning gut to be able to absorb fat from the diet. As vitamin D is fat soluble it cannot be found in foods which don't contain fat. People who may be affected include those with Crohn's disease and liver disease.

Those who live further away from the equator or work indoors because:

- They are exposed to less sunlight.

Those on cholesterol lowering drugs such as statins because:

- Cholesterol is required to make vitamin D

Dietary sources of Vitamin D

- Cod Liver Oil: one tablespoon contains approximately 1,400 international units. In the shorter months - from October until March - I would recommend two tablespoons daily for anyone with a neurodegenerative disease or who belong to the susceptible groups already mentioned above.

- Cooked salmon: three ounces contains about 450 international units
- Beef liver: three ounces contains about 40 international units
- Egg yolk: one large, 40 international units[19]
- Irradiated mushrooms: three ounces, 35 international units.

As you can appreciate, it is difficult, if not impossible to take in up to 4000 IU's of vitamin D, daily, through diet. Useful sunlight can only be found between the months of May until the end of September when it comes to the synthesis of vitamin D.

As vitamin D is a fat soluble vitamin it must be taken with a little fat in order for it to be absorbed.

Inhibitors of Microglia

---

[19] *Irradiated mushrooms have been left out in the sun and absorb ultra violet rays.

Microglia are immune system cells that are one of the brain's defences when infection crosses the blood brain barrier. They do a remarkable job once activated but do have a tendency to get out of control and become a major player in auto immune diseases of the brain such as motor neuron disease.

The group of antibiotics known as the tetracycline's are known to inhibit microglial activation especially minocycline. In spite of this knowledge, minocycline is not routinely prescribed for those where microglia are known to play a part in the pathology of neurodegenerative diseases.

The good news is that **Resveratrol** – a substance found in the skin of red grapes – is known to inhibit microglial activation. Most people will have heard of resveratrol in connection with red wine. Indeed, the love of wine so often attributed to the French people may be a major protective factor not only for preventing cardiovascular disease but for neuroprotection, too.

Resveratrol appears to restore the integrity of the blood brain barrier preventing harmful immune molecules from infiltrating the brain tissues. In addition, resveratrol helps remove beta amyloid plaque from the brain.

It also has excellent anti-oxidant effects but these, unfortunately, do have low bio availability.

On the negative side, resveratrol has been found to have bi-phasic effects. This means it has can have both positive and negative impact on neural tissue. However, given its diverse benefits, it is being looked at as a potential treatment for neurodegeneration.

Although resveratrol is found in good quantities in red wine there is another potent flavonoid contained in red wine that has a powerful therapeutic effect on dementia. This flavonoid is known as quercetin and we shall return to it later.

Non-steroidal anti-inflammatory drugs (NSAID's)

This particular class of drugs has been found to significantly decrease the likelihood of being diagnosed with Alzheimer's disease, thus providing evidence of inflammatory processes underpinning this disease.

Common NSAID's include:

- Ibuprofen
- Aspiring

- Celebrex
- Diclofenac
- indomethacin

NSAIDS block prostaglandins. Prostaglandins are a family of chemicals that are produced in the body. They have a number of vital functions. They promote inflammation that is necessary for repair of damaged tissues.

When inflammation becomes chronic, it serves no useful purpose. It can cause further damage to tissue with ensuing pain. Therefore, NSAIDS can be useful in dealing with low lying subclinical inflammation.

However, NSAID's have a number of unwanted side effects. They can damage delicate kidneys and reduce prostaglandins that help protect the stomach lining, among others.

NSAIDS may be useful in the short term but there are also many foods that contain salicylates that also help to suppress inflammation. It is to these that we will turn to next.

Salicylates

Salicylates are chemicals found in plants which have pain- relieving, anti-pyretic and anti-inflammatory properties. They are naturally occurring in many fruit and vegetables and help to protect plants from being attacked by fungus. Salicylates are also found in aspirin.

Studies have shown that aspirin might reduce the risk of ALS, and the benefit might be more prominent for older people.[20] The reason is thought to be because older people are more likely to take larger doses daily. Another study indicates that treatment with NSAID's, like aspirin, can restore brain cell production as well as lower levels of beta-amyloid by reducing inflammation. The latter is good news for those with Alzheimer's disease and other diseases which are fuelled by inflammation. While the number of neurons may increase, it does not necessarily mean that function is restored. The restoration of function has to be learned and is an entirely different process.

---

[20] Nov. 14 issue of *Science*, Dr. Steven Paul and researchers from the drug maker Eli Lilly and Co.

Other studies have shown similar findings in that salicylic acid-based treatments may help prevent excessive neuronal loss in neurodegenerative diseases. As such salicylates may have some therapeutic value in treating or preventing many neurological diseases.

Aspirin has been found to be very effective at reducing free radicals by mopping them up in a very efficient manner. As free radicals injure and damage tissues then clearly reducing them is beneficial.

There are a number of downsides to taking aspirin and salicylates. Some of the side effects of aspirin are the potential for indigestion, gastritis and ulcers. Salicylates may cause allergy type symptoms, in susceptible people. These include

- Asthma like symptoms – wheezing and trouble breathing
- Headaches
- Nasal congestion
- Changes in skin colour
- Itching, skin rash and hives
- Swelling of the hands, feet and face
- Stomach pain

However, if aspirin and salicylates are not a problem then they can be included as a treatment to reduce the inflammation found in neurodegeneration.

Foods containing high amounts of salicylate are:

- **Fruit**

Blackberry, blackcurrant, apricots, blueberry, dates, grapes, orange, pineapple, plum, strawberry, prunes, raspberry and sultana

- **Vegetables**

Chilli peppers, courgette, green olives, peppers, radish and water chestnut

- **Seeds and nuts**

Almonds, peanuts with skins on

- **Honey**

Herbs, spices and condiments

Coconut oil, olive oil, basil, bay leaf, caraway, chilli powder, nutmeg, vanilla essence

Buffered Soluble Aspirin, similar to Alka Seltzer, can be home made

2 uncoated aspirin

8 oz soda or sparkling water

1/2tsp baking soda

Juice from a wedge of lemon

This buffered soluble aspirin is not appropriate for those on a sodium restricted diet.

.

DMSO

Dimethyl sulfoxide (DMSO) is the by-product of papermaking. It is a drug that benefits human cells, tissues and organs and helps in bringing systemic cellular function back to health.

DMSO is able to control swelling, banish inflammation, kill bacteria, viruses and fungi or at least slow down their ability to multiply allowing the immune system to adequately respond to any infection. It has been found to open blocked sinuses within a few minutes of application to the nostrils.

DMSO is able to bond strongly with hydroxyl groups. It is a scavenger of hydroxyl radicals that are major ions in pain syndromes such as arthritis. Hydroxyl ions are known to break down synovial fluid and cartilage. However, DMSO also works on other areas where inflammation is present. Atherosclerosis and neuroinflammation respond to DMSO. This is good news for those with Alzheimer's disease and vascular dementia.

DMSO is reputed to have sixteen major therapeutic uses with no known contraindications. One of its properties is its ability to inhibit cholinesterase.

Cholinesterase is an enzyme that breaks down acetylcholine. Acetylcholine is the neurotransmitter that helps form memories and assists learning. It is found in lower levels in those with Alzheimer's disease so inhibiting the enzyme that helps break it down has therapeutic properties.

As DMSO attacks the disease and not just the symptoms, users find that they need to use DMSO less often and in lesser quantities as time goes on. Further, DMSO does not have to be applied directly to the injured part, if this is not appropriate. It's pain relieving and anti-inflammatory properties are effective if applied topically some distance away from the injury.

It is recommended that DMSO is prescribed by a registered health practitioner but it is available without prescription. Many individuals who self-prescribe apply it to clean skin, four times daily for twenty minutes at a time. It is then washed off.

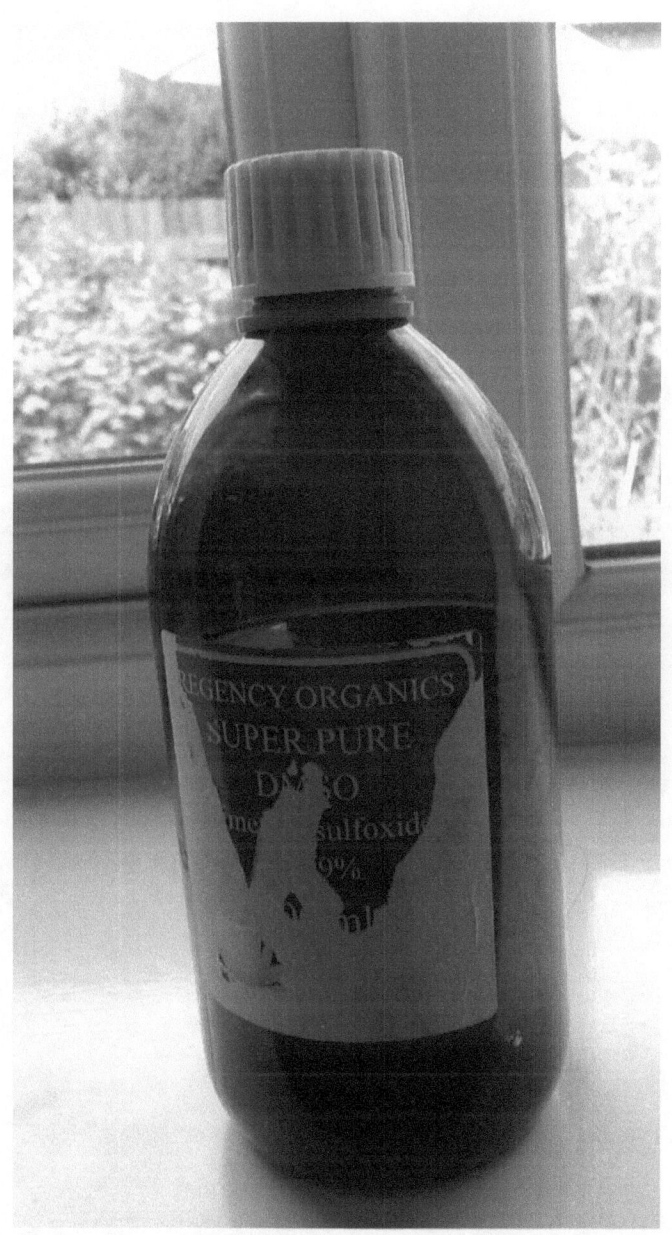

Quercetin

Quercetin is a flavonoid that is found in many fruit and vegetables but is specifically found in red onions, apples and red wine.

Food	Amount
Grapes, black (100 g)	2.17 mg
Red Raspberry, raw (100 g)	3.58 mg
Nectarine, whole (100 g)	0.11 mg
Broccoli, raw (100 g)	1.80 mg
Red onion, raw (100 g)	1.80 mg
Black tea, infused (100 ml)	1.13 mg
Red wine (100 ml)	1.14 mg

[21]

---

[21] https://www.integrativepro.com/Resources/Integrative-Blog/2017/Quercetin-Food-Compared-Supplementation

The administration by injection of 25mg/kg every 48 hours for murine participants showed that quercetin decreases:

- Extracellular beta amyloidosis
- Tauopathy
- Astrogliosis
- Microgliosis

In the hippocampus and the amygdala.

As these terms aren't in general use, it may be useful to define them now.

Tauopathy – clumping of tau protein due to disease

Extracellular beta amyloidosis – the build- up of abnormal protein. In this case, the brain.

Astrogliosis – an abnormal increase in the number of astrocytes due to disease

Microgliosis – the proliferation and activation of microglia in the brain. These are concentrated around amyloid plaques. Microgliosis is a prominent feature of Alzheimer's disease.

As quercetin was also found to induce improved performance on learning and spatial memory tasks[22],

---

[22] https://www.ncbi.nlm.nih.gov/pmc/articles/PMC4387064/

the findings suggest that this flavonoid reverses the characteristics of Alzheimer's disease in murine models.

Quercetin has the ability to cross the blood brain barrier and is protective against atherosclerosis. It is also protective against ischaemia which is a restriction in blood supply that supplies nutrients and oxygen to tissues.

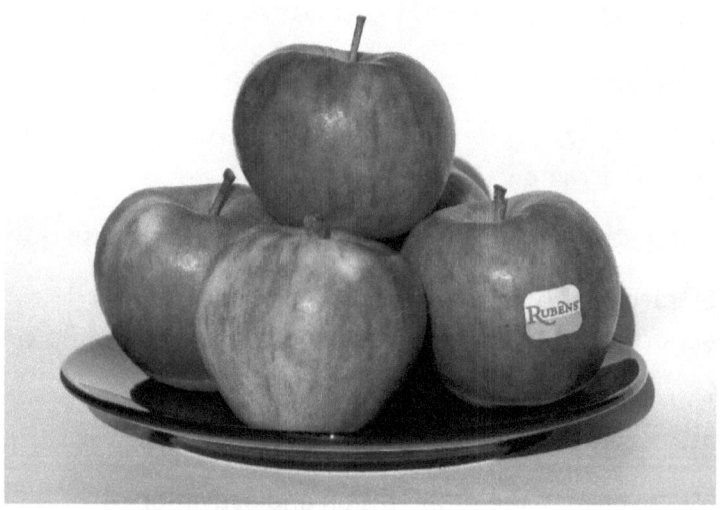

Apples contain good amounts of quercetin

In spite of government advice to eat five a day of fruit and vegetables, it is doubtful whether this amount would supply the amounts of quercetin necessary to maintain good neural health.

74

Quercetin has indirect benefits for protecting neural tissue. We have already discussed that anti-cholinergic medications are associated with pathological changes, in neural tissue, that are characteristic of Alzheimer's disease. Some of these over the counter medications are anti-allergy medications that are used to treat the symptoms of hay fever and other allergies.

Mast cells are generally responsible for the distressing side effects associated with allergies such as streaming eyes, stuffy noses, itchy throats and sneezing.

Quercetin has well documented mast cell stabilising activity. As such, it can attenuate the symptoms of allergic reactions without the concerns over the damage to neural tissue that can be caused by taking anti-cholinergic medication.

Useful Information

Preclinical Stage of Alzheimer's Disease	Characterised by • Abnormal protein deposits found in amyloid plaque • Neurofibrillary tangles • Healthy neurons stop functioning and begin to lose their connections in the hippocampus and entorhinal cortex

KNOWN – or likely - CAUSATIVE FACTORS of DEMENTIA and REMEDIES

Pre-clinical and Clinical Stages Included

Known or likely causative factors of neuropathological changes in Alzheimer's disease and vascular dementia	Remedy
Poly unsaturated omega 6 oils	Remove omega 6 vegetable oils from the diet. Use stable saturated fats such as lard and butter that do not cause inflammation Increase amount of docosahexanoic acid found in oily fish. Fish oil has been found to elevate a protein - LRll that prevents the formation of amyloid beta protein.
Sugar	Reduce sugar as much as possible.
Trans fat	Remove all trans fats from the diet. In some countries they are banned
Arachidonic acid as it • Increases inflammation • Activates tau	Omega six poly unsaturated fatty acids found in most vegetable oils should be removed from

kinases which increases phosphorylation of tau • Increases beta amyloid (in murine models)	the diet. Look at labels in processed foods. 'safe' oils are olive oil and fish oil Use saturated fats as in advice for poly unsaturated omega 6 oils above
Bacteria	Keep zinc levels at optimum levels 11mg for men and 8mg for women daily. Zinc activates T lymphocytes which prevent infection.in vascular and Alzheimer's disease.
Low co-enzyme Q10 levels – • Co-enzyme Q0 increase Kappa Beta levels which prevents release of substances that increase inflammation • Q10 protects mitochondria as beta amyloid protein is toxic to mitochondria	Take Q10 supplements
Low selenium levels – found to be reduced in those with Alzheimer's disease	Take Brewer's yeast or eat two Brazil nuts daily
Beta Amyloid (build up	• Eat fish as it

causes tau tangles)	elevates a protein that prevents beta amyloid
	• Drink coffee as caffeine lowers beta amyloid levels
	• Eat foods containing quercetin as this reduces beta amyloid and taupathy
	• Eat foods with curcumin in as this reduces the build-up of beta amyloid by breaking it down. Quercetin is able to cross the blood brain barrier.
	• Eat foods that contain resveratrol as this helps remove amyloid beta protein from the brain.
	• Increase foods

	containing zinc in the diet as zinc binds to amyloid beta and redirects its assembly to amorphous aggregation
Low grade inflammation due to free radicals	• eat plenty of fresh fruit and vegetables and whole wheat food. Fresh fruit and vegetables contain antioxidants and salicylates which reduce inflammation • eat plenty of foods containing glycine that help prevent microglial activation
Reduced levels of acetylcholine due to • lack of nutritional substances to make acetylcholine • too much cholinesterase (the enzyme that breaks down acetylcholine	• eat plenty of foods that contain glycine (found in gelatine and gelatinous products) and choline which help form acetylcholine • use olive oil as the monounsaturated fatty acid helps produce and

	release acetylcholine • Use 99% pure DMSO diluted with distilled water as it inhibits the breakdown of cholinesterase
chronic microglial activation	eat foods that contain resveratrol
low levels of DHA omega 3 – individuals with low levels of DHA either have Alzheimer's Disease or have a high risk of being diagnosed with it	eat plenty of oily fish or take cod liver oil
Copper status – high levels lower the clearance rate of amyloid beta protein from the brain to the blood	Zinc inhibits the absorption of copper. Increase foods containing zinc.
Zinc deficiency – zinc binds to beta amyloid so that there are fewer reactive oxygen species zinc changes shape of amyloid beta protein to a less toxic shape	Eat more foods containing zinc.
Statins – as they dysregulate the mevalonate pathway which is involved in: • Co-enzyme Q10 production	Follow the steps found in the book 'Why you live longer with higher cholesterol levels.'

• and is also involved in the synthesis of Kappa Beta • use of statins has been proven to increase the risk of infection • A high percentage of cholesterol is found in the brain and is necessary for brain health as well as reducing inflammation.	

The connection between thiamine deficiency and Alzheimer's disease

Thiamine is part of the vitamin B complex. It was the first of the B complex to be discovered so is known as vitamin B1. Thiamine is required for the correct functioning of every cell in the body. It acts as a cofactor to a number of enzymes in the pyruvate dehydrogenase enzyme complex which is a critical step in carbohydrate metabolism.

Research has focussed on the reduced metabolism of glucose as a potential cause of cognitive decline and Alzheimer's disease.

In a 2019 paper by Bridget M Kuehn MSJ, she commented that:

Areas or patterns of reduced glucose metabolism are often seen in brain scans of patients with Alzheimer disease and other dementias. Now, a growing body of evidence suggests that glucose hypo metabolism may be more than just a biomarker on brain scans: it may be a key player in dementia pathology.[23]

23

At an annual meeting of the Society for Neuroscience, a number of research team presented data on various mechanisms that hindered brain energy metabolism in Alzheimer disease.

The paper does not state whether thiamine was part of the presented data. I believe that if it wasn't then a serious error has been made.

Thiamine deficiency goes by the name of beriberi. It's signs and symptoms are diverse reflecting the fact that it is required in every cell of the body. However, to clarify what I intend to talk about, it is better to focus on the three main types of beriberi. The signs and symptoms often overlap. It would be rare if they were confined to one area of the body. Nevertheless, symptoms may appear worse in one of the types of beriberi, over the other two.

The three forms are:

Dry beriberi (involving the central and peripheral nervous system)

Wet beriberi (involving the cardiovascular system)

Gastrointestinal beriberi (involving the gastrointestinal tract)

---

https://www.sciencedirect.com/science/article/abs/pii/S0361923005004338

For the main part I will focus on   dry beriberi since the symptoms it causes are the ones that cause most concern in matters of cognitive decline.

Dry beriberi has many symptoms but the main ones are recognisable by those who care for those with Alzheimer's disease.

- Vomiting

- Erratic eye movements known as nystagmus

- Mental confusion and speech difficulties

- Tingling

- Pain

- Difficulty walking and a tendency to lose balance

- Loss of sensation in hands and feet

- Weak limbs, difficulty getting up from a chair, may   eventually result in paralysis of lower limbs.

- Losing the thread of a conversation

- Forgetting where you've put things

- Finding it difficult to multi task

- Brain fog

Of course some people may recognise some of these in themselves. They may be informed by health professionals that it is part of the ageing process. It is not. It is a sign that there is a deficiency somewhere that needs correcting as the sooner it is, the less damage there is to repair.

Now, to return to the subject of impaired glucose metabolism. This is clearly a problem found in diabetics who are at higher risk of thiamine deficiency. Research does show that they often have a deficiency of thiamine which is compounded by those who are prescribed Metformin. Metformin degrades thiamine by inhibiting the Human Thiamine Transporter TTHR-2. These transporters are found in the kidneys, liver, intestine, placenta, central nervous system and muscle among other tissues   so play an important part in the overall health of the body.

There are other problems connected with the administration of Metformin but this is not the only cause of a thiamine deficiency.

Leaving aside the obvious cause of malnutrition which appears rife in today's society where there are more food fads than ever before – most of them not guaranteed to increase health but designed to increase profit – elderly people do not absorb nutrients as well as they did when they were younger. Often their appetites reduce - or their motivation to cook healthy food   does - especially if they have no-one but themselves to cook for.

The PPI's – antacids – and diuretics are more or less guaranteed to result in dementia at some point. The former prevents the absorption of valuable nutrients like thiamine and its activator magnesium, and the latter just flushes every vital nutrient out of the body including thiamine and its activator, magnesium.

Tea, coffee, high carbohydrate diets, raw fish (shellfish and sushi, for example) quercetin – which appears to be very popular with many who do not realise that ample amounts exist in onions, leeks, garlic and other members of the onion family as well as a wide variety of vegetables – also inhibit thiamine.

Thiamine is indeed a vulnerable B vitamin – more so than many of its siblings. As it is water soluble, it easily leaches into cooking water, is destroyed by heat and storage.

The foods we used to eat – lightly cooked liver, malt, malted milk, yeast extract, pork, peanuts and nuts in general, have largely fallen out of favour - and to our detriment.

Alzheimer's disease – and many other neurodegenerative disorders like Parkinson's disease, multiple sclerosis, vascular dementia, motor neuron disease - appear to come about due to a defect in the intracellular metabolism of glucose of which thiamine deficiency must now take centre stage.

It is well known that when thiamine deficiency occurs then there is build-up of the amyloid beta plaques characteristic of Alzheimer's disease. When therapeutic doses of thiamine are administered to the patient then the amyloid beta plaques dissolve and are removed from the system.

In a recent communication I had with someone who administered thiamine to their grandmother who had Alzheimer's disease, the granddaughter reported that after 3 weeks the grandmother had become 'more in the middle' and had more lucid moments than non-lucid ones. It is early days yet. The full effects of thiamine may not be seen for 6 months, maybe even more if neurodegeneration has been severe. However, there will be some effects felt even within hours of taking thiamine. Sometimes, these can be quite subtle but some have reported within 3-7 days:

I can walk up the steps without holding onto the rail and having to put both feet on the same step. (2 weeks of taking thiamine).

The ability to walk down the centre of the steps without placing feet on the same step or holding onto a rail. (one week's thiamine)

5 good nights' sleep in a row from day 1 of taking thiamine when I have not slept properly for two years.

Depression – long standing – lifted. (three days therapy)

Suddenly got up, after not being motivated to do anything for weeks, and cleaned the house. (3 days of thiamine).

More energy, more focus (3 days of therapy with thiamine).

More sociable, far less social anxiety and it's improving by the minute.

Able to speak coherently, was unable to find the words I wanted prior to taking thiamine.

I have regained my love of cooking – previously I used to forget the recipe, forget what stage I was at and where the ingredients were in the cupboard.

Far less irritable – my husband is going to make sure that I never run out.

This is only a few of the many comments I have had about the huge benefits that thiamine has had.

As well as dissolving beta amyloid plaques, thiamine has also proven to be useful in Lewy Body Dementia (LBD) which is characterised by hallucinations and abnormal deposits of alpha-synuclein protein. The deposition of this protein can result in hallucinations, disturbed and distressing behaviour, movement and thinking disorders as well as problems with mood.

Brandis et al 2006 in his paper on **Alpha-synuclein fission yeast model: concentration-dependent aggregation without plasma suggested that an increase of cellular thiamine could reduce alpha- synuclein concentration and thereafter alpha-synuclein aggregation without plasma toxicity membrane localisation or toxicity.** *J Mol Neuroscience 2006;28179-191*

Found that both the aggregation and concentration of this protein could be reduced.

It seems to me that when you have a deficiency of a nutrient which causes the symptoms of well-known dementias which resolve when sufficiency of the nutrient is restored through therapeutic intervention, then the deficiency – in this case thiamine in the form of dry beriberi) and the disease – in this case known as Alzheimer's disease – are one and the same.

How would gastrointestinal beriberi fit into the picture? Even without all the meds which are known to cause constipation and other digestive upset – Alzheimer's (as well as other neurodegenerative disorders) are characterised by constipation. It is uncomfortable and distressing – especially more so for a patient who cannot verbalise their discomfort. In those with early stage Alzheimer's disease – through my work in the past – it was noted that they reported long standing and intractable constipation in spite of a diet with plenty of fibre, fluid and exercise.

Of course, thiamine deficiency also affects the gut. Thiamine is needed for the release of hydrochloric acid from the gastric cells. Without enough acidity in the stomach, the upper valve cannot close leading to regurgitation of stomach contents, indigestion and heartburn.

The lower valve will not open leaving food sitting heavily in the stomach. Bloating and abdominal distension ensue and, of course, there is also constipation.

It is rare to find a patient with Alzheimer's who does not have diabetes or some cardiovascular problem for which they will be given a package of meds which do little for their health. True, it may provide immediate relief but it does not address the underlying deficiency that is causing all the problems. Sadly, the package of medicines given out will probably need more medicines to be prescribed   to cope with the side effects. And so it goes on. Elderly people with all the wisdom of their years   and a wonderful and long retirement to look forward to, are found to be bewildered, drooling and living their last years out often in places that cannot and do not give them the love, care dignity and attention that they deserve.   Indeed, if they were not deficient in this vital nutrient then it is quite likely they would still live independently in their homes, contributing all their valuable skills to the community, bouncing their grandchildren on their knee, cooking for the family and taking their proper place in society.

The Recommended Daily Intake (RDI) of thiamine is just 1.4mg. There is clearly something grossly wrong with this. It is paltry. It does not address anywhere near, the needs of people.

Thiamine has not been found to have any upper tolerable limit. This means it has not been found to be unsafe in even large doses of 4g (4000 mg). It is not known to interact with any prescribed or over the counter medication. It is a safe vitamin.

Doses are variable depending on the needs of the individual. Some people do very well on 100mg – indeed many brands of this standalone vitamin start at 100mg. Some people take doses of 300mg and find their symptoms resolve at this amount.

Those with neurodegeneration may start at 500mg three times a day. If there is no effect whatsoever after one week then it can be increased. If a slight anxiousness occurs, then stop the dose for a couple of days then use a slightly lower dose on a daily basis. You will soon find the right level.

There are many forms of thiamine or its derivatives like benfotiamine. The latter is fat soluble and is said to create higher levels in the body. However, there is some doubt whether it crosses the blood brain barrier so is of no use to people with a neurodegenerative disorder.

I have used a number of the other types of thiamine and cannot see that there is anything between them. Indeed, when researching I have found that different research papers will promote different types of thiamine over the other.

The most common one and the cheapest appears to be thiamine mononitrate and I have found it to be excellent. For 120 days' supply of one tablet of 100mg at little over £5.00 then I would suggest that anyone with any form of dementia, try increasing their thiamine intake through food and supplement form. Magnesium is the activator so it needs to be taken with a little magnesium at the same time. Sometimes, a diet rich in magnesium does not need supplementation but if you are not sure, then this is the best way forward.

Thiamine costs very little and could make the world of difference,

As the B vitamins work together synergistically, then it is prudent to take a good vitamin B complex alongside the stand alone thiamine. You will notice that the amount of thiamine in the complex will be very small and is nowhere near enough to address chronic neurodegenerative disorder.

At the moment, I have only heard positive results from those who have either taken high dose thiamine themselves or administered it to their loved ones. I am confident that this will continue.

We have learned that Alzheimer' s disease is a 'new' disease that has coincided with the introduction of 'healthy foods to the developed world's diet. These foods are, in fact, highly inflammatory. Further, they have replaced the omega 3 oils from our diets - including DHA - that are known to help remove plaques from brain to blood.

When white bread was introduced – and quickly became popular – the major source of B complex that is vital for removing the toxic homocysteine was removed from our diets. In addition, thiamine was removed and even though it was added back it may not be in a bioavailable form.

Sleep disorders are rife. We have more street lights, more light from screens, more noise pollution. The environment is never still. There is little difference between night and day now. It is no wonder that stress and anxiety are words that we hear pouring out of people's mouths nowadays.

As we have already seen, sleep appears to be the body's time to clear out toxic material including beta amyloid which it transfers from brain to blood.

Stress also plays a part. During stressful events the stress hormone rises helping to facilitate the release of glucose into the bloodstream. This starts the furring up process – atherosclerosis -found in those with dementia, particularly of the vascular type.

The increase of the availability of over the counter anti-cholinergic medication is a major cause of concern given that pathological changes characteristic of Alzheimer's disease are seen with limited or sporadic use of these medications.

I have oft stated – and I cannot repeat it enough – that diseases rise and fall depending on the prevailing environmental factors at the time. We introduce new foods. medications into our diet and as we relinquish others our potential for different disease states is changed.

If we live in colder climates, our body fat will increase to protect us from the cold. If we ingest pro inflammatory oils, then we are potentially setting up the potential for future cardiovascular disease and other inflammatory disorders that are currently rife in society.

Obesity is an inflammatory disorder. People are becoming unhealthier and it is not all down to lack of exercise. It is partly a disorder of the range of foods – and thus nutritional substances - that are available to the public at any specific moment in time. With inflammation comes swelling and pain. Individuals appear to be suffering from low grade systemic inflammation.

Even if you are aware that omega 6 vegetable oils create inflammation and avoid using it, it is ubiquitous in food. It appears in ice cream, bread, commercially produced cakes and biscuits, among others. In fact, there are very few commercially produced foods that do not contain omega 6 oils. Even the margarines produced from sunflower oil are advertised as being healthy even though they are inflammatory in nature.

Some people do appear to be able to cope with the increasing amounts of inflammatory foods in our diets. However, others do not. The difference is explained by genetic factors. However, no one knows which genetic mix they have inherited. Even if they do not have a genetic propensity for dementia, the highly explosive pro inflammatory foods that we are presented with nowadays will exert their effect on some other more vulnerable part of the body. This could include joints or heart or kidneys, to name but a few.

It may take a while for individuals to realise that saturated fat is not the enemy. Indeed, saturated fat has been shown to lower any inappropriately high levels of cholesterol. Further, as a stable fat it does not generate free radicals freely.

Individuals do not appear to be able to differentiate between what is hype about food, in the pursuit of profit, and what is reality. Cookery lessons, which also educated about the food groups, vitamins and minerals are not part of the general curriculum. Therefore, we have lost the knowledge to be able to evaluate claims about new foods appearing on the shelves.

Vegetable oils look 'cleaner' than saturated fat. White bread looks better than the heavy and unrefined grain bread that used to be eaten. We eat 'healthy' flapjack little realising that it contains pro inflammatory vegetable oil. Our national fish and chips are now cooked in it instead of the dripping that was once used.

Our meat and two veg have now become spaghetti or pizza. The latter two have little in the way of antioxidants.

Breakfasts that used to consist of a couple of boiled eggs and slice of wholemeal toast with butter have now become a breakfast muffin and a glass of bottled water. Eggs are an essential food for healthy brains as is wholemeal bread. Eggs contain lecithin and this a major dietary source of choline which we have already found is vital for brain health as it may reduce the rate of progression of dementia.

It should be clear by now that our diets have changed dramatically over the last hundred years and, as they have done so, there has been a surge of 'new' diseases that have not been noted before in the population. Our present diets appear to lean towards degenerative changes in the brain. What is clear is that there is a huge rise in the dementias and this is predicted to rise over the next couple of decades unless the causative environmental factors are dealt with.

Vegetable oils, white bread and flour and our changing meals are so much a part of our lives that change for the population as a whole, if it does come, will be slow and painful. Nevertheless, there is nothing to stop each individual from making those changes for themselves and their families right now.

About the Author

Lynne Noble was born in 1953 in Huddersfield, West Yorkshire. From a very early age, Lynne showed an interest in nutrition and genetics avidly reading any books that she could get her hands on at the time.

Initially, Lynne studied orthopaedics but events led her to work with the elderly mentally infirm. Here, her interest in neurodegenerative disorders and pain syndromes developed.

Lynne undertook rigorous programmes of study, completing her Cert Ed., (FE) BSc (Hons) and Adv. Dip Education simultaneously before moving onto her M.Ed.

From there she took further demanding programmes in Human Nutrition, Pharmacology, Neuroscience, Genetics and Immunology. During this time, she was given many prestigious awards for her academic work. It was noted then that Lynne was not afraid of tackling difficult subjects.

She began her law degree but ill health prevented her from pursuing this. However, in this time, she moved from being a foster parent to adoptive parent.

She has been instrumental in setting up projects in the community for disadvantaged groups.

She is a member of the Guild of Health Writers.

Now retired, she lives in a picturesque village in West Yorkshire with her husband. She enjoys gardening, watching her husband bowling and researching.

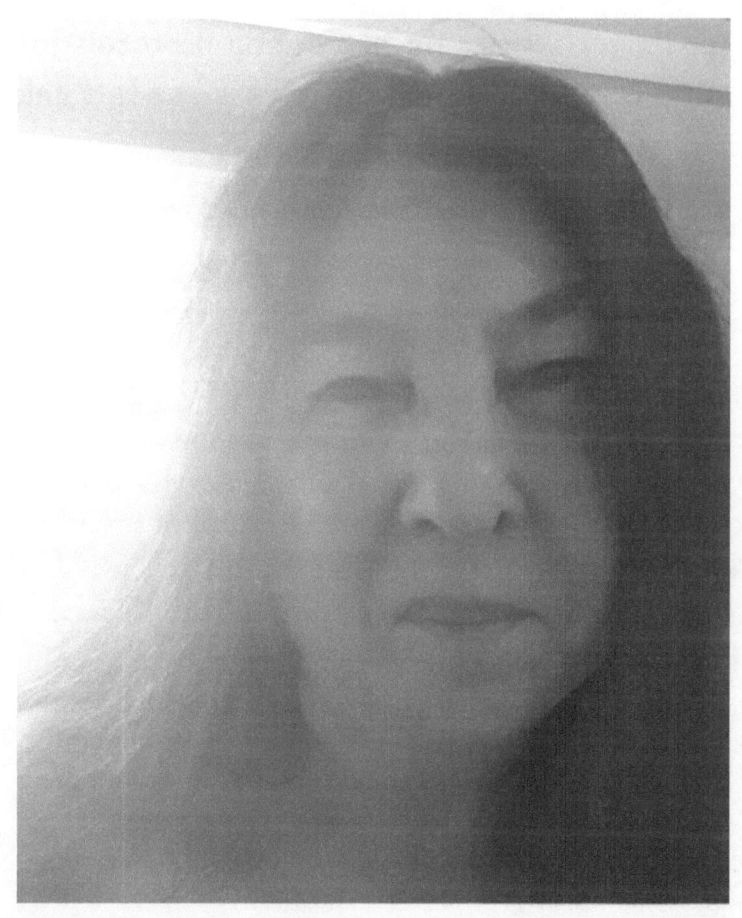

Author Lynne Noble at home

https://quintessentiallylynne.weebly.com/nutritional-medicine.html

for longer articles on health and protocols for various medical conditions please use this link below

https://www.buymeacoffee.com/lynnedmnobl

The MND Diet by Lynne D M Noble is a comprehensive diet handbook that looks at the possible causes of neurodegeneration and how nutrition can respond to the challenges of neurological conditions. It is a useful addition to the information contained in this book.

The book Why you   Live Longer with Higher Cholesterol Levels explores the benefits of cholesterol and how it is necessary for memory and overall health. The book also reveals the dark side of taking statins and how taking statins cause increase the risk of being diagnosed with cardiovascular disease and disorders of the brain. It offers solutions – through bespoke diet – of lowering any potentially harmful cholesterol that exists.

A percentage of the royalties from the sale of these books are used for charitable purposes. One such charity that has benefitted is The Exodus Project.

The Exodus Project

My first introduction to the far reaching impact of The Exodus Project occurred when I was travelling around Cawthorne in one of their buses, visiting gardens. A young lad was happily munching on a sandwich. He looked up briefly, pointed to the driver and said,' He's my second dad, he is,' then he returned to his sandwich without further comment

Such remarks are often very telling and so I arranged to meet Jackie Peel and Martin Sawdon, at the charity's premises in Barnsley. They set up the Exodus Project 20 years ago. They moved into their current premises – a redundant Methodist church - in 2010.

Both Jackie and Martin have been youth workers in their church. Martin worked in housing for the homeless in addition to working in learning disabilities services in institutional settings.

The work that the Exodus Project undertakes is of paramount importance to the communities it serves. These were former mining communities which became disadvantaged after pit-closures. Currently about 400 children attend mid-week activities from Monday to Thursday inclusive. These activities include dance, drama, craft, music, sports and games. In addition, there are weekend camps, cycle treks, outward bound activities, bowling and swimming. The children are taught valuable life skills including how to cook and bake. It is all about teaching children how to fulfil their potential and learn skills they will be able to pass onto the next generation.

The grounds, once overgrown, have been turned into a play- and camping - ground. A miniature railway is in the process of being installed.

Martin and Jackie have developed a unique model in that The Exodus Project goes beyond dispensing services. They are keen to build up relationships with the whole family and not just the child that attends the mid- week clubs. In addition, once children have reached the age of fourteen, they are invited to help out with the younger groups as junior volunteers. Once they reach the age of eighteen, they become adult volunteers. This model provides a constant supply of help from individuals who have benefitted already from attending such groups.

The building is large and inviting. It is decorated with bold colours and has comfy seating. It is a real home from home; a haven for families who have been disadvantaged by the closure of the life force of its community.

Martin and Jackie have clear ideas about how they wish to develop the Exodus Project but the lottery funding which they benefitted from is no longer available. Sadly, they have had to close two of their clubs due to lack of funding. This decision wasn't taken lightly. They do have two charity shops which raises some money and they obtain some funding from outside organisations for the use of their facilities. However, this is clearly not enough to keep their clubs, weekend activities and building going to cater for the ever growing number of children who are benefitting from the work being undertaken here. Neither does it allow for future development.

Exodus do have a Just Giving page which can be found here if you wish to help further their work https://www.justgiving.com/exodus

In addition, you can keep up with activities on their Facebook page here

https://www.facebook.com/search/top/?q=the%20exodus%20project%20barnsley&epa=SEARCH_BOX

If anyone wishes undertake an event like The Three Peaks - or run a marathon to raise funds for Exodus - then Martin or Jackie would be pleased to hear from you. This will enable their vital work in the community to continue. Contact them through their website to be found on www.exodusproject.org.uk.

www.ingramcontent.com/pod-product-compliance
Lightning Source LLC
Chambersburg PA
CBHW051352280526
45784CB00007B/2928